100 Metabolic Workouts

Phil Bennett

"If you want to be a CHAMPION You need to Train like one "

~GSP

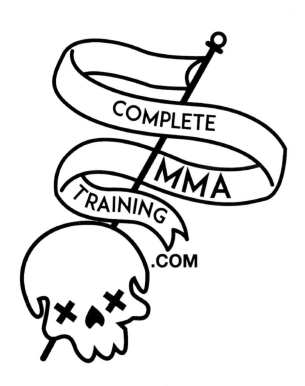

Disclaimer

The information presented within this book is in no way intended as medical advice or to serve as a substitute for medical counselling. The information presented herein should be used in conjunction with the guidance of your physician. Always consult your physician before starting this program as you would with any exercise or nutritional program. If you choose to abstain from seeking the consent of your physician throughout this program, you are agreeing to accept full responsibility for your actions. By starting the workouts contained within this manual, you recognize that despite all precautions on the part of Complete MMA Training, there are inherent risks of injury or illness which can occur due to your use of the aforementioned information and you expressly assume such risks and waive, relinquish and release any claim which you may have against Complete MMA Training or their respective affiliates as a result of a any future physical injury or illness incurred in connection with, or as a result of, the use or misuse of your program.

All rights reserved. No part of this program may be reproduced (by any means) without the expressed written consent of Phil Bennett and Complete MMA Training.

This information is being provided for educational and informational purposes only.

Please be sure to consult your physician before starting this or any program. There is an inherent risk with physical activity. Phil Bennett or Complete MMA Training cannot be held responsible for any injury that may occur during participation with this program.

Copyright 2015 Complete MMA Training

The World of Metabolic Workouts

The days of steady state cardio are over. Plodding along on a treadmill at a slow, meaningless pace is a thing of the past. If you are looking to burn fat, increase your overall athleticism and look and feel great, metabolic circuits are for you.

What exactly is a Metabolc Workout?

Metabolic workouts are all about intensity and efficiency. They are short, often no more than 20 minutes of work. The number one benefit of metabolic training though is the fat burning potential. This is done by raising your post exercise oxygen consumption or EPOC for short. In its simplest form, EPOC means that you will continue to burn calories and fat even after your workout is over. The more intense your workout, the more you raise your EPOC. This means you can be burning fat all day long with a workout that is just 20 minutes of 100% intensity training.

You may be wondering "how is it possible to replace a long jog with a short circuit?" You wouldn't be alone in thinking this.

It was once believed that only aerobic exercise (the long steady state jog) increased cardiovascular health. Numerous studies are now showing that anaerobic exercises (short intense exercises) condition your heart to the same, if not higher levels than aerobic exercises do. Perhaps the most famous study comes from Dr. Izumi Tabata.

The study found that athletes that completed an intense burst of anaerobic sprinting experienced higher levels of VO2 max improvement than the control group, who performed 60 minutes of moderate exercise.

Benefits of this kind of Training

8 reasons you need to do these workouts regardless of whether you are a seasoned athlete or just looking to get fitter.

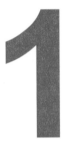

Higher Levels of Athleticism

Performing even the most basic of exercises with high levels of
intensity in a circuit will effectively raise your heart rate and increase your overall levels of athleticism.

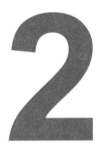

Get Results Quickly

This short, intense style of training wakes up your metabolism. This in turn will increase your cardio levels, build lean muscle and burn fat.

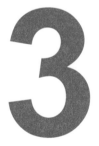

Lean Muscle Gains

Your body is an amazing machine. When you push its limits, it will respond as needed. In this case that means more HGH (human growth hormones) to keep up with the work load and power outputs.

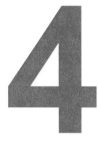

The Mental Push

Mental toughness is a huge aspect in achieving the things you want.
Exercise is no different. You must push yourself as hard mentally as you do physically to complete the workouts. If you are an athlete performing these routines as finishers to your main workout, then this mental toughness you develop will carry over into your sport, forcing you to work as hard as you can until the end.

A Break from the Norm

Exercise at the end of the day should be fun and something you enjoy. Plodding along on the treadmill or road is not fun, it's tedious and frankly quite boring. This kind of training is interesting, challenging and never the same twice. It may be tough while you are doing it, but it's an enjoyable kind of tough.

Calorie Burn

It's possible to burn anywhere from 300-650 calories per workout based on your height, weight, gender, fitness levels and intensity. Not bad for something that is less than 30 minutes!

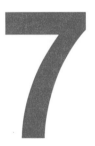

The EPOC

I mentioned earlier the benefits of EPOC. The workouts in this book are short and intense in nature, setting you up nicely for the EPOC afterburn. The benefits of EPOC have been shown, in many cases, to continue burning calories up to 36 hours after completing the routine. If that isn't enough incentive to put in 100% effort, then I don't know what is.

The Challenge

These workouts are hard. They will feel like torture when you are grinding through them. You have to constantly remind yourself of the benefits and just how little time the workouts take.
Challenge yourself, beat your former performance and in no time you will look, feel and perform exactly like you want to.

Who is this Book for?

This book is a guideline for anyone who wants to lose weight, get fitter and become more athletic overall. It's for those who are short on time, those who work full time with a family and have no time for the gym. It's for full time moms with kids who get very little time to exercise. It's for full time students who have no cash for a gym membership.

It's also for those who want to push their conditioning levels to new limits. The exercises contained within this book have all been used by me and the fighters I train. After any practice is over, the group will perform one of the circuits listed. When the circuits provided are performed at the end of workouts or practice, they are designed to make sure you have burnt every single bit of energy you have left. They become an exercise in not only conditioning, but also in mental toughness and satisfaction.

So, if you are looking to drop a little weight, don't have the time or cash for a gym membership or you are a competing athlete looking to push your conditioning levels, then there is something in this book for you.

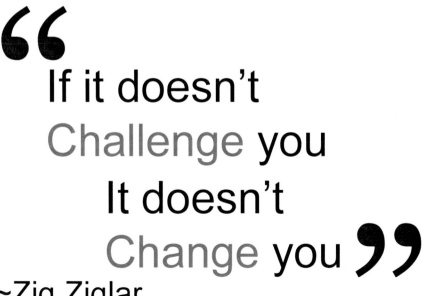

" If it doesn't Challenge you It doesn't Change you "
~Zig Ziglar

10 Ways to get the Most out of the Workouts

1 Check in with your physician first. This is the case with any new program and this one is no exception.

2 Always make sure you know the correct form on any exercise. Form is not only key to getting the most out of any exercise, but it is the way to prevent injuries. Consult a professional who can coach you in the correct form.

3 Never go into a workout hurt. Training with an injury is just going to slow down your healing and potentially make things worse. Feeling tight or working through DOMS is perfectly fine however.

4 Be sure to scale the exercises to your level of fitness. Going too heavy too soon is going to hurt you. Be realistic, make proper progressions and you will be a beast in no time.

5

Be constantly aware of signs of overtraining. Rest is as much a part of training as going hard is. If you are feeling super beat up, stressed, struggling to sleep, fatigued, then you need a rest. Make sure you always eat well and healthy, rest well, sleep well and practise stretching and soft tissue work.

6

Progress at a clever rate. Don't assume you can go from beginner to beast in one week. Training strength and conditioning takes time. Just like learning a new technique. Consistency and small gains are key.

7

If you follow this program 100% and put in your maximum effort, you will burn fat and increase fitness levels.

8

Performing a warm-up is a must. Never underestimate a quality warm-up.

9 I touched on this earlier, but it needs repeating. Do not start this program if you are nursing an existing injury. Rest, rehab and get yourself to full health before you begin.

10 If you put 100% effort into the training for that day, you will never need to perform more than one circuit. If you feel you have the energy for a second, you didn't push yourself enough on the first.

" The Beginning is the most Important part of the work "

~Plato

Workout Guidelines

Frequency: How many days a week do you need to train?

This is really up to you as an individual. In a perfect world four times a week would be ideal. This isn't always an option though. Even just twice a week will make a huge difference to your health, attitude and appearance. As I mentioned earlier if you are training in a sport or martial art, fitting one workout in at the end of practice will be incredibly beneficial to your performance. Depending on your schedule, fitting in a workout should be pretty easy because they are all very short in nature.

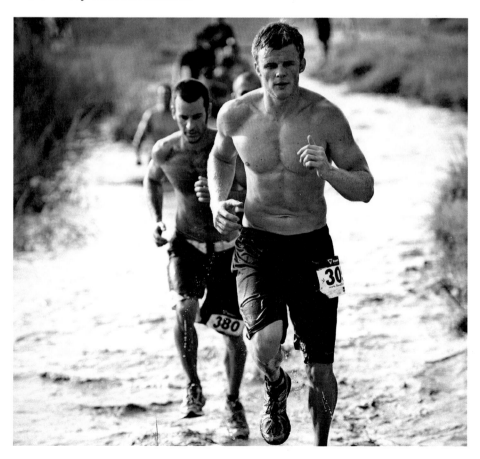

Intensity: What effort are you expected to give?

Simply, this is the amount of work you put in, in the time given. If you are given 30 seconds to perform an exercise, you need to be performing as many as you possible can fit in within the time frame. If the exercise is not time-based, but rather repetition-based, then each repetition needs to be 100% of your focus and effort.

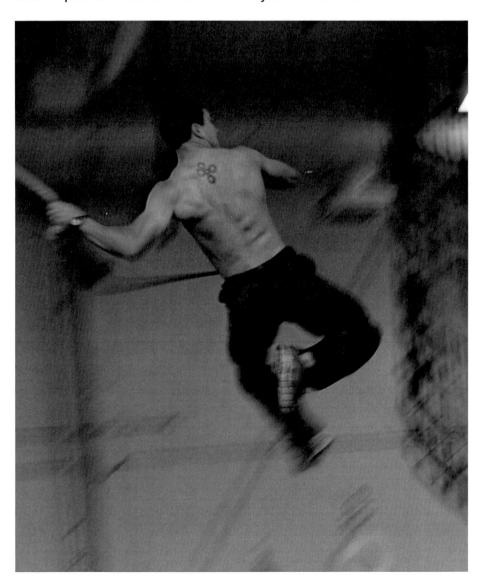

Time: How long do these workouts take?

Depending on your current level of fitness, or the level of the exercise, the routines take anywhere from 2 minutes to 30 minutes. On average you are looking at a 20 minute routine including the warm-up.

Equipment: What do you need to perform these workouts?

As I mentioned earlier, all the workouts contained within this book require just your body weight. No other resistance or weight is needed. Trust me, this will be enough!
For certain exercises you will need something to hang from. This could be a pull-up bar, a door attachment pull-up bar, a soccer goal post or a tree. Whatever will work as long as you can safely hang from it.
The only other requirement for certain exercises is an open space. A garden, sports field or open field will work well for this. This isn't the case for every workout though. Many of the workouts contained within this book can be done in a single room with enough space hold your arms out to the sides. I am 6ft 6 and frequently perform these workouts in hotel rooms, so really you have no excuse there!

One Final Point

It's inevitable that you will tire during these workouts. They are tough and brutal and designed to get you to PUSH your limits. That said though, never let your form suffer because of fatigue! There is nothing cool about terrible form. Swallow your pride and go to easier variations of the exercises if your form is suffering. Adjusting the exercises in this manner will avoid potential   injury.

The Warm Up

Warming your body up is essential. A comprehensive full-body workout will not only increase your body temperature, but it will also increase mobility and coordination, and prepare your body for the workout ahead. Your brain will get fired up and your central nervous system will get prepped.

Never skip over your warm up!

It is essential to remain healthy, prevent injuries and increase your performance.

Foam Rolling

The first part of your warm up is a self-myofascial release. This is the fancy term for a self-massage. This can be done with a foam roller, a hard ball, such as a lacrosse ball, or your own hands. You will apply pressure to specific parts of your body to remove knots, trigger points and scar tissue that accumulates in your body. By doing this self-massaging, you will eventually restore your muscles natural length and reduce lingering pains. This is a fairly quick process where you want to spend a few minutes rolling over your calves, quads, groin, hips, glutes, lats and upper back. Go over roughly 10 rolls on each of these parts, sticking on any particularly tight or tender spots. Once you are thoroughly rolled, you are onto the dynamic part of the warm up.

"Before anything else, Preparation is the key to Success"

~Alexander Bell

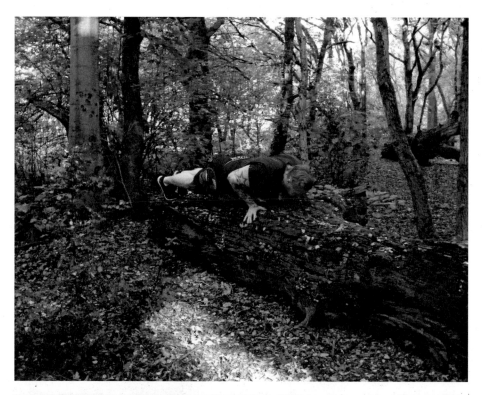

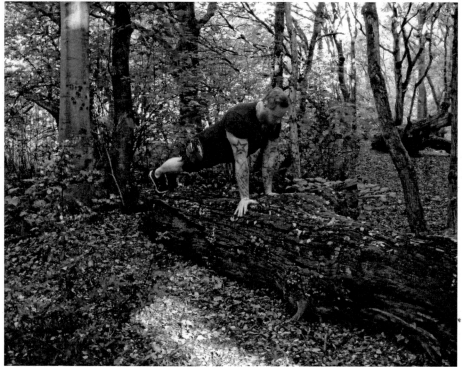

Dynamic Warm Up

1 Jump Rope x 3mins

2 Big Arm Circles x 10 forward, 10 backwards

3 Front to Back Leg Swings x 10 each leg

4 Cross Body Leg Swings x 10 each leg

5 Lunges x 5 each leg

6 Squats with Arms Overhead x 10

7 Inch Worms x 5

8 Push-up x 10

9 Jumping Jacks x 25

10 A. Jog Forward/ Jog Backwards x 15 yards

B. Side Shuffle x 10 yards each way

C. High Skips x 15 yards

" It's hard to beat a person that Never Gives Up "

~Babe Ruth

Here's the good stuff…

Remember train HARD, but SAFE

1 Brutal Basics

Prisoner Squats x 30 seconds
Push-ups x 30 seconds
Rest x 30seconds

Repeat this pattern for a total of
5 rounds.

2 Race to 100 Burpees

As the name implies, start a timer and
stop it once you have completed 100
full burpees.

3 Push-up Madness

Wide Grip Push-ups x 12 reps
Push-ups x 9 reps
Diamond Push-ups x 6 reps
Clap Push-ups x 3 reps

Rest for up to 2 minutes and repeat for a total of 3 times.

4 Air Born Insanity

Burpee x 2 reps
Jump Squat x 2 reps
Clap Push-up x 2 reps

Complete as many rounds as possible in 10 minutes.

5 Isometric Killer

Wall Handstand x 30 seconds
Plank x 30 seconds
Rest x 30 seconds

Repeat this pattern for a total of 5 rounds.

6 Posterior Power

Glute Bridge x 10
Superman Raise x 10
Deep Squat x 10

Repeat this circuit 4 times with minimal rest between each.

66 # Suffer the pain of
Discipline
or suffer the pain of
Regret 99

~Jim Rohn

7 Pulling Madness

Inverted Row x 50 total reps
Chin-up x 40 total reps
Pull-up x 30 total reps
Dead Hang x 2 total minutes

Rest as needed. Just finish the reps prescribed above.

8 Tricep Torture

Diamond Push-up x 30 seconds
Dips x 30 seconds
Bodyweight Tricep Extensions x 30 seconds

Repeat the pattern above for a total of 5 rounds.

9 Slow Strength Push-ups

Each push-up will take 20 seconds to complete.
5 seconds hold at the top
5 seconds lowering
5 seconds at the bottom (1 inch from the floor)
5 seconds rising to the top.

Complete as many as possible in 10 minutes.

10 Crawl Sprint

Bear Crawl x 25 meters
Sprint Back x 25 meters

Complete as many rounds as possible in 15 minutes.

11 Feel the Burn!

Wall Squat x 30 seconds
Squat x 30 reps

Repeat as many times as possible in 10 minutes.

12 Boxer Style

Burpees x 10 reps
Simulated Jump Rope x 100 reps

If you have access to a jump rope,
perform 100 rope turns each round.
If you do not have access to a rope,
simulate the motion alternate foot
hopping as if you were jumping rope

Complete 10 rounds for a total of 1000 rope turns
and 100 burpees.

13 Jumping Power

Box Jump x 2
Broad Jump x 4
Squat Jump x 8
Rest 60 seconds

Repeat for a total of 5 rounds.

14 Ladders

Push-ups x 10,9,8,7,6,5,4,3,2,1
Squats x 10,9,8,7,6,5,4,3,2,1
Dips x 10,9,8,7,6,5,4,3,2,1
Pull-ups x 10,9,8,7,6,5,4,3,2,1

Perform these in which ever order you choose. If you start with the
pull-ups for example you must complete all the prescribed reps
before going onto the next exercise.

15 CoreCrusher

Mountain Climber x 30 seconds
Plank x 30 seconds
Double Crunch x 30 seconds
Hollow Hold x 30 seconds
Rest 60 seconds

Repeat for a total of 3 times

16 Gassers

Set up cones at 10 meters, 20 meters, 30 meters, 40 meters and 50 meters.

Sprint to the first cone, and then back to the start line.
Immediately sprint to the second cone and back to the start line.
Then to the third cone and back.
Forth cone and back.
Finally to the fifth cone and back.

This is one giant set. Rest 2 minutes and repeat 3 times total.

"When you are going through hell, keep Going"
~Winston Churchill

17 Death by Burpee

Burpees x 1 rep, then 2 reps, then 3 reps up to 20 reps, then back down, 19 reps, 18 reps until you get back down to 1 again.

This is a total of 400 gruelling reps.

18 Like a Climber

Side to Side Pull-ups x 4 each side
Pull-up Hold x 10 seconds

Repeat as many times as possible in 15 minutes

19 Hand Walks

Inch Worms x 5
Handstand Wall Walks x 3

Repeat for a total of 4 times.

20 Fighters Fatigue

Shadow Box x 30 seconds
Sprawls x 30 seconds
Drop Steps x 30 seconds
Clinch Knees x 30 seconds
Shadow Box x 30 seconds
Repeat for 8 rounds total.

21 Animal Madness

Bear Crawl x 20 seconds
Crab Walk x 20 seconds
Monkey Hops x 20 seconds
Rest 30 seconds
Repeat for a total of 10 rounds

22 Burpee Sprints

Burpee x 10 reps
Sprint 20 meters
Burpee x 10 reps
Repeat for 10 rounds total

"30 Minutes of working out is just 2% your day. NO EXCUSES"

23 Spiderman!

Spiderman Push-up x 6 each side
Spiderman Crawl x 10 meters
Broad Jump x 5

Repeat for a total of 5 rounds

24 Singles

Pistol Squat x 3 each leg
One arm push-up x 3 each arm

Complete the reps on the left side of your body before going onto the reps for the right side of your body.

Complete for as many rounds as possible in 10 minutes.

25 Big 500

Squat x 100
Burpee x 100
Push-up x 100
Pull-up x 100
Dip x 100

No guidelines, rest as you need, perform as you like.
Just get the 500 reps finished.

26 Around the World

Bulgarian Spilt Squat x 30 seconds
Thai Push-ups x 30 seconds
Russian Twists x 30 seconds
Rest 30 seconds

Repeat for a total of 6 rounds

27 No Crunches Here

Flutter kicks x 50
Mountain Climber x 50

Rest as little as possible. Repeat for a total of 10 rounds

28 Boxers Endurance

Jab Cross x 60 seconds
Alternating Uppercuts x 60 seconds
Alternating Hooks x 60 seconds
Rest 30 seconds

Repeat for a total of 5 rounds

29 100 Steps

Walking Lunges x 100 total reps per leg
Step ups at Mid Thigh Height x 100 total reps per leg

Rest as needed, just complete all the reps prescribed.

30 Hardcore100

Burpee/Pull-up combo x 20
Clap Push-up x 20
Pistol Squat x 20 per leg
Tuck Jump x 20

Complete the reps as fast as possible.

31 Tabata Sprints

Sprint Flat out for 10 seconds
Walk for 20 seconds

Repeat this 10 times.

32 200 Reps of Hell

100 Judo Push-ups
100 Tuck Jumps

Complete the reps however you want, just get the reps done.

"Fitness is not about being better than someone else. It's About being better than You used to be"

~Brett Heobel

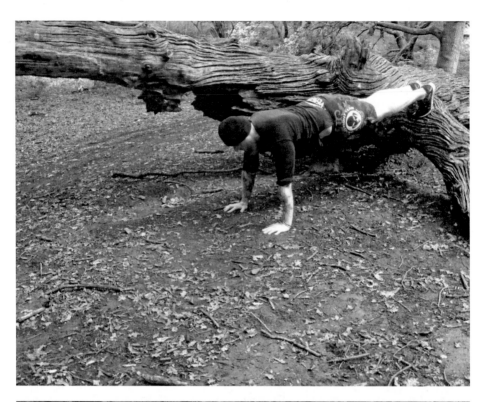

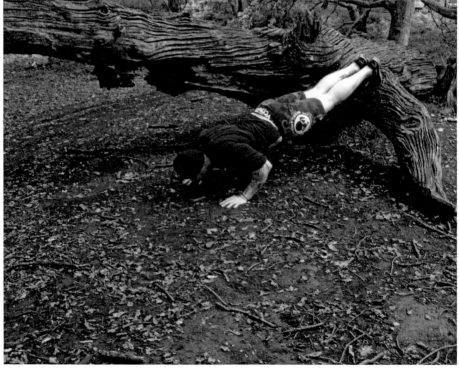

33 Epic Shoulders

Pike Push-up x 10
Handstand Push-up x 5
Handstand Hold x 30 seconds
Rest 60 seconds

Repeat 4 times total.

34 BJJ Endurance

Chin-up Holds x 20 seconds
Shrimp x 20 seconds
Technical Get-ups x 20 seconds
Egg Beaters x 20 seconds
Sit through x 20 seconds
Rest 30 seconds

Repeat for a total of 5 rounds

35 One Move Murder

Burpee with Push-up at the bottom and
a Tuck jump at the top x As many as
possible in 8 minutes.

36 Lung Buster

Hill Sprint x 50 meters
Hindu Push-up x 10

Complete 4 rounds total.

37 Legs don't stop

Run 400 meters
Walk 100 meters
Run 300 meters
Walk 100 meters
Run 200 meters
Walk 100 meters
Run 100 meters

38 Sprinters Delight

10 x 10 Meter Sprints-
Rest 20 seconds between each.

5 x 100 Meter Sprints-
Rest 60 seconds between each.

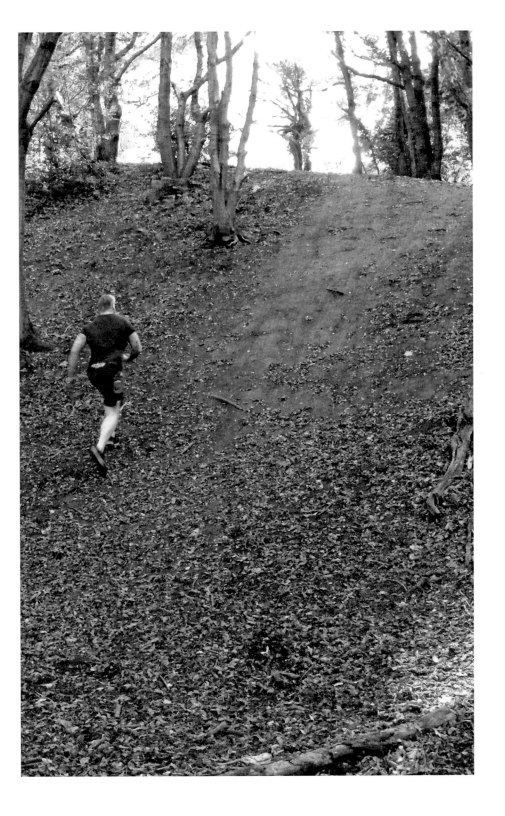

39 Animal Madness 2

Alligator Walk x 30 seconds
Duck Walk x 30 seconds
Kangaroo Hop x 30 seconds
Rest 30 seconds

Repeat for a total of 5 rounds.

40 Finger,Hand and Wrist Strength

Finger Push-ups x 5
Knuckle Push-ups x 10
Finger Push-up Hold x 10 seconds
Knuckle Push-up Hold x 20 seconds

Complete 3 rounds in total, resting well
between each.

41 Bear Necessities

Bear Crawl for a total of 10 minutes.

Do this is in as many sets as you want, resting whenever you want. Just get a total time of 10 minutes bear crawling.

42 Walk, Run, Sprint

Walk x 60 seconds
Run x 60 seconds
Sprint x As long as possible.

Continue this cycle until you have completed 8 rounds.

43 Lateral Thinking

Lateral Step-ups x 10 each side
Lateral Lunges x 10 each side
Burpees with lateral Jump x 4 each side
Rest 60 seconds

Repeat for a total of 3 rounds.

44 As many as you can

Pull-ups x As many as you possibly can
Push-ups x As many as you possibly can
Squats x As many as you possibly can

> **66** **Motivation** **is what gets you started. Habit is what keeps you going.** **99**
> ~Jim Ryan

45 Fighting against your Mind...

Wall Squat x failure
Inverted Row top position hold x failure
Back Bridge x failure
Plank x failure
Hollow Hold x failure
Push-up Bottom Position Hold x failure
Cliff Hanger x failure

Rest well between each exercise and be sure to fight against your mind telling you to stop. Hold each for as long as physically possible.

46 Inverted World

Hold a Handstand for a total time of 8 minutes.

47 99's

Tuck Jumps x 33
Burpees x 33
Broad Jumps x 33

Perform the reps as you like. Just complete the reps prescribed.

48 4 Way Core

Plank x 30 seconds
Left Side Plank x 30 seconds
Right Side Plank x 30 seconds
Superman Hold x 30 seconds

Repeat for a total of 3 times.

49 Load of L's

L-sit Chin-up x 8 slow reps
L-sit Hold x failure
Hanging Leg Raise x 8 slow reps

The key here is performing the reps slow, increasing your muscles time   under tension. This circuit will only need to be done 2 times.

50 Row and Go

Inverted Rows x 12
Burpee x 12

Perform as many rounds as possible in a 10 minute period.

51 The Dive Bomber

Complete a total of 250 Divebomber push-ups

52 MMA Conditioning

Jab Cross Sprawl x 60 seconds
Hip Escape/Shrimp x 60 seconds
Shadowbox x 60 seconds
Simulated Armbar from Mount x 60 seconds
Drop shots/Duckwalks x 60 seconds
Rest 60 seconds

Challengers complete 3 rounds, Champions complete 5 rounds.

53 HoppingMad

Frog Jump x 100 meters

Rest as long as you need and complete 4 lengths in total.

54 Against the Clock

On the minute Sprint 75 meters. Rest the remaining time left in the minute.

Repeat this pattern until you cannot beat the clock anymore.

55 Even More Sadistic Burpees

Begin flat on your back. Stand and perform a burpee with a push up at the bottom and a broad jump at the top.

Complete as many reps as possible in 5 minutes.

56 Runners Delight

Run as far as you can in 60 seconds
Walk for 60 seconds

Repeat for a total of 5 times.

57 Fighters 100

Straight Punches x 100
Clinch Knees x 100
Front Kicks x 100
Elbows x 100

"It's not who you are that holds you back. It's who you think you're not. "

~Denis Waitley

58 Traditional Tabata

Flat out High Knee Sprint in place
x 20 seconds
Light Shadowbox x 10 seconds

Repeat the pattern for a total of 8 times.

59 Feeling on Fire

Ab Bicycle x failure
Plank x failure
Mountain Climbers x failure

Rest 60 seconds and repeat for a total of 5 times.

60 Defend to Attack

Sprawl to Jumping Knee x 100 total reps per leg

61 Bye Bye Legs

Squats x 200
Burpee x 100
Tuck Jump x 75
Frog Jump x 50
Broad Jump x 25

Perform in any order you choose. Just complete the reps listed.

62 Ground Fighter

Sit Throughs x 20 per side
Hindu Push-ups x 20

Complete as many rounds as possible in 10 minutes.

63 The Archer

Archer Push-ups x 5 each side
Archer Pull-ups x 3 each side

Complete as many rounds as possible in 15 minutes.

64 Pistoleros

Pistol Squats x 50 per leg

"Being Challenged in life is inevitable Being defeated is Optional."

~Roger Crawford

65 Monkey Fitness

Monkey Hops x 30 seconds
Chin-ups x 10
Monkey Hops x 30 seconds
Pull-ups x 5
Monkey Hops x 30 seconds
Dead Hang from bar x failure

Rest as needed and repeat for a total of 3 times.

66 Furious Box Jumps

Burpee to Box Jump x 2
Box Jump x 4
Burpee x 6
Box Jump x 4
Burpee to Box Jump x 2

Rest as needed. Repeat for a total of 3 times.

67 Hold and Explode

Wall Squat Hold x 30 seconds
Squat Jump x 5
Push-up Bottom Hold x 30 seconds
Clap Push-up x 5
Rest for 60 seconds

Repeat for a total of 5 rounds.

68 Gymnast Inspired

Pseudo Planche Lean x 10 seconds
Handstand Hold x 20 seconds
Hollow Hold x 30 seconds

Rest as needed and repeat for a total of 5 times.

69 Slowing Time

Pull-up that takes a full 10 seconds to get to the bar
Hold for 3 seconds at the bar
Take a further 10 seconds to lower to a Dead Hang
Dead Hang for a further 3 seconds

Complete 10 reps total.

70 Push and Crunch

Diamond Push-up x 10
Crunch x 40
Push-up x 20
Crunch x 30
Wide Grip Push-up x 30
Crunch x 20
Rest 60 seconds and repeat for a total of 3 times

71 Single Leg Hell

Cossack Squat x 50 total each leg
Pistol Squats x 50 total each leg

72 Ancient Martial Arts

Horse Stance Hold x 10 Minutes Total

> "To be a Champ you have to believe in yourself when nobody else will."

~Sugar Ray Robinson

73 Simple but Effective

Diamond Push-up x 10
Chin-up x 10

Rest as needed. Complete 10 rounds in total.

74 Banana Style

Hollow Hold x 30 seconds
Superman Hold x 30 seconds

Rest 30 seconds and repeat for a total of 4 rounds.

75 Dead Man Walking

Walking Lunge x 100 meters

Rest 60 seconds and repeat for a total of 3 times.

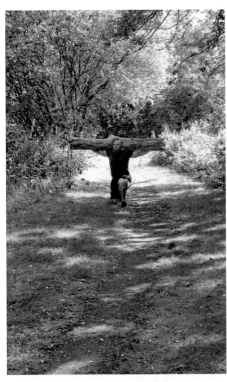
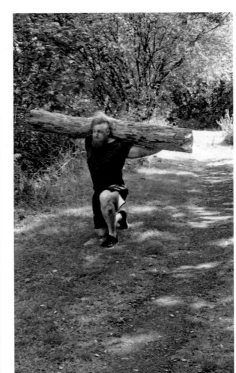
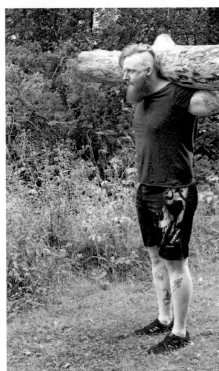
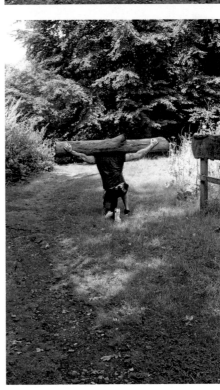

76 Handstand Power

Handstand Hold x 30 seconds
Handstand Shoulder Taps x 10
each shoulder

77 Submission Special

Kimura Sit-up x 10 each side
Guard Triangle attack x 10 each side

Repeat for a total of 5 rounds.

78 Tigers and Dragons

Tiger Push-ups x 50 total
Dragon Flag x 30 total

79 Pushing from all Angles

Handstand Push-up x 3
Pike Push-up x 6
Decline Push-up x 9
Push-up x 12

Rest 90 seconds and repeat for a total of 3 rounds.

80 Hop, Skip, Jump

Lateral Jumps x 30 seconds
Bounds x 30 seconds
Burpee x 30 seconds

Repeat for a total of 5 rounds.

81 How does Spiderman do it?

Spiderman Crawl x 50 meters
Broad Jump x 50 meters

Rest as needed. Repeat for a total of 3 times.

" The meaning of life is not simply to exist.

But to move ahead, to...

CONQUER **"**

~Arnold Schwarzenegger

82 Mental Test

400 meter run
50 Squats
300 meter run
50 Squats
200 meter run
50 Squats
100 meter run
50 Squats

83 Hindu Strength

Hindu Squats x 250 total
Hindu Push-ups x 250 total

84 Towel Grip Circuit

Towel Grip Pull-ups x 3
Towel Grip Chin-up x 5
Towel Grip Inverted Row x 7
Towel Isometric Squeeze x 10 seconds
Rest 60 seconds and repeat for a total of 3 times.

85 Rocky Special

Jump Rope Sprint x 100 rope turns
One Arm push-up x 3 each arm
Repeat for 5 total rounds.

86 Isometric Hell

L-sit x failure
Tuck Planche x failure
Plank x failure
Right Side Plank x failure
Left Side Plank x failure
Bridge x failure
Hollow Hold x failure

Push yourself on each exercise. You are only performing each once, so make it count!

87 Dirty 30

Dragon Flag x 10
Hanging Leg Raise x 10
Lying Leg Raise x 10

Rest 90 seconds and repeat for a total of 3 times.

88 Football Special

Up Downs x 20 seconds
Lateral Shuffles x 20 seconds
10 Yard Sprint

Rest 60 seconds and repeat for a total of 5 rounds.

89 The Commando

Commando Pull-ups x 50 each side total.

90 Giant Arms Circuit

Diamond Push-ups x 12
Bodyweight Tricep Extension x 10
Push-up x 10
Chin-up x 8
Bodyweight Bicep Curl x 6
Rest 60 seconds and repeat for a total of 3 times.

66 The Greatest pleasure in life is doing what people say you cannot do **99**

~Walter Bagehot

91 Shadow Wrestling

Stay in stance, move in all directions.
Sprawl every 10 seconds.
Take a shot every 15 seconds

Keep this going for a total of 8 minutes.

92 Heart Pounder

Burpee x 10
Squat x 1
Burpee x 9
Squat x 2
Burpee x 8
Squat x 3
Burpee x 7
Squat x 4
Burpee x 6
Squat x 5
Burpee x 5
Squat x 6
Burpee x 4
Squat x 7
Burpee x 3
Squat x 8
Burpee x 2
Squat x 9
Burpee x 1
Squat x 10
As Fast As Possible.

93 The Grinder

Push-ups x 2 minutes
Squats x 2 minutes
Pull-ups x 2 minutes
Burpee x 2minutes

94 Hanging Gymnast

Skin the Cat x 3
Muscle-up x 1

Rest as much as needed. Repeat for a total of 5 times.

95 Muay Thai Endurance

Skipping Knee Twists x 30 seconds
Close Grip Chin-up x 30 seconds
Alternating Single Leg Knee Bridge
x 30 seconds
Spiderman Push-up x 30 seconds
Rest 30 seconds
Repeat the circuit for a total of 6 times.

96 Total Strength and Agility

Alternating Pistol Squats x 100 total
Side to Side Push-ups x 100 total
Side to Side Pull-up x 50 total
Handstand Hold x 5 minutes total

97 97 Core Hell

Flutterkicks x 97
Plank Push-ups x 97
Mountain Climbers x 97
Hollow Hold x 97 seconds

Rest as needed. Just get the reps done.

98 Power Glutes

Glute Raise x 15
Deep Squat x 12
Reverse Plank x 60 seconds
Rest x 60 seconds

Complete 5 rounds total.

99 Advanced Push and Pull

Handstand Push-up x 5
L-sit Pull-up x 5
Decline Push-up x 5
One Arm Inverted Row x 2 each arm

Complete as many rounds as possible in 15 minutes.

100 Centurion

Tuck Jumps x 100
Burpee x 100
Push-up x 100
Inverted Row x 100

Rest as needed. Just get the reps done.

"What doesn't kill you makes you Stronger"

~Nietzsche

Frequently asked questions

When should I use these workouts?

These workouts are in no way meant as a full workout program. They are, however, one hell of a resource for those who are short on time, those looking to push cardio limits and those looking for a quick workout for fat loss.

If you are looking to complete any of the routines within this book, I urge you to scale them to your level of fitness. The level of intensity, however, remains the same. Regardless of the level of the exercise, you must put in 100% effort and intensity. Limit your workouts to once per day, which with 100% effort, will be more than enough.

For coaches and athletes, I strongly recommend you end your sessions with one of the workouts within this book. Attacking the routines in this book as a workout finisher is an amazing way to destroy your training session. It will improve cardio levels, burn fat, build muscular endurance and the mindset alone will help you get more results in the main part of your training session.

Are these routines just for fat loss?

Nope. While the routines found in this book will ultimately get you leaner, they will also get you stronger and more athletic. There are workouts out of the 100 that will challenge you even if you are a seasoned athlete. By working with this style of training, you are going to lose weight, build muscle and get fitter, regardless of your current level of fitness.

How should I use these workouts?

You should use the workouts in this book as a guide rather than a program. If you are looking for a workout with little time and no equipment, there is something in here for you. Set aside a small amount of time (30 minutes is enough) and complete one of the 100 contained in here. Keep things consistent. Be sure to do this at least twice a week, if possible, or four times to see maximum benefits. Challenge yourself. Choose a new workout each time you train. Don't stick with the same few you have become familiar with. Push yourself and break through your limits.

Coaches and athletes have the added benefit of competition. Finish the training session with a group challenge. This added competition element will push you and your athletes harder and to new levels of fitness.

Even though I mentioned earlier that it's best to mix things up and use as many of the workouts within this book as possible, it's inevitable that you will end up repeating one you have previously done. Keep note of your performance last time you completed the challenge, like the time it took you, the reps you managed to do and how you felt. It's these simple gauges that will tell you of your progress.

I can't think of reasons not to train.

I'm glad! The workouts within this book are the perfect excuse breakers. If you want to get fitter, leaner and stronger, it's your responsibility to find the time. I understand that not everyone has hours a day to train, but luckily some of the routines in this book are as short as 5 minutes work! If you are short on time these workouts are fast and best of all, effective.

"20 Years from now you will be more disappointed by the things that You Didn't Do Than by the ones You Did Do."

~H. Jackson Brown Jr

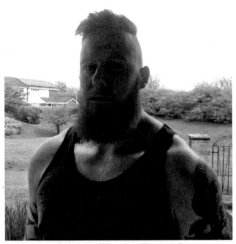

About the Author

Phil Bennett is a strength coach from the UK who primarily trains combat athletes. He has a particular, gym-less style of training that utilizes objects provided by nature as well as odd object like kettlebells, sandbags, kegs, ropes, chains and the like. His primary focus as a coach is combat/human performance, mental toughness and real world strength.

Make sure you head over to CompleteMMATraining.com for more training advice, unusual workouts, strength training, MMA and combat sport specific strength and just generally how to become a bad-ass.

While you are there make sure you sign up for the weekly newsletter and as a gift for signing up you get instant access a comprehensive grip training eBook to train your way to an unstoppable vice like grip.

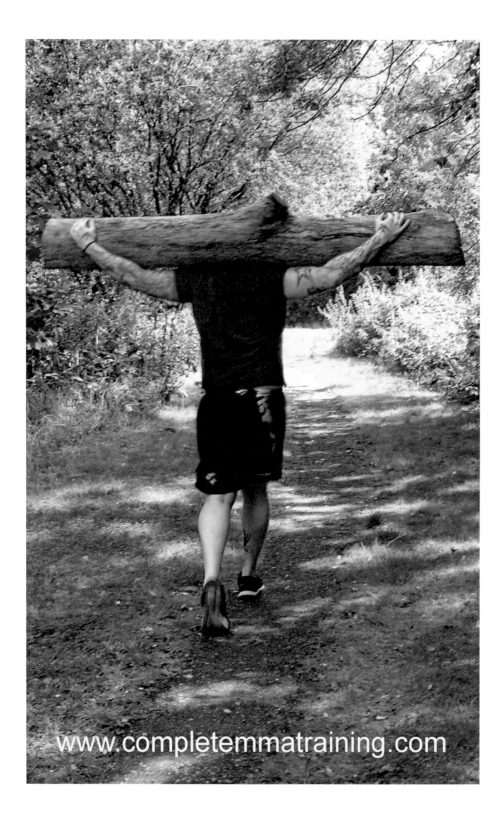

Made in United States
North Haven, CT
18 March 2023

34242760R00042